TUBERCULAR
MIASM
TUBERCULINS

D1736640

TUBERCULAR MIASM TUBERCULINS

Explained and Simplified

Dr. FAROKH JAMSHED MASTER
M. D. (Hom.)

Co-authored By
DR. FIRUZI DABU
B.H.M.S. (BOM.)

B. JAIN PUBLISHERS (P) LTD.
USA — EUROPE — INDIA

TUBERCULAR MIASM TUBERCULINS

First Edition: 1992
Second Edition: 1992
8th Impression: 2013

Published by Kuldeep Jain for

B. JAIN PUBLISHERS (P) LTD.
1921/10, Chuna Mandi, Paharganj, New Delhi 110 055 (INDIA)
Tel.: +91-11-4567 1000   Fax: +91-11-4567 1010
Email: info@bjain.com   Website: **www.bjain.com**

Printed in India by
JJ Imprints Pvt. Ltd.

ISBN: 978-81-319-0272-1

DEDICATED

TO

Dr. B.E. Patell,

B.Sc., D.M.S. (Cal)

It is for your spirit in Homoeopathy that I write this book as well as to Rukshin my beautiful daughter, and Mahaziver my new born daughter.

PREFACE

Nosodes are remedies derived from diseased tissues and secretions containing the specific organism of the disease.

The only way to use a nosode is to prove it on the healthy, like any other drug, and note its symptoms in the recognised way of provings.

By potentising a nosode one develops their latent dynamic forces; hence, they should be prescribed as conscientiously as any other remedy.

All the nosodes have their own characteristics and it is important for a student to study from all reliable sources.

To begin with let us revise the meaning of constitution, Miasm, and its representation from Psora to Syphilis.

By constitution I mean diathesis or dyscrasia inherent in an individual.

By Miasm I mean a stigma or taint.

According to Dr. K.N. Kasad, miasm can be represented from Psora to Tubercular to Sycosis and Syphilis.

Each miasm has its own general characters but we

frequently find combinations in patients; it is for the Homoeopath to recognise these inherent tendencies. The recognition of such traits in patients before they become parents, would remove constitutional encumbrances in future offspring.

After the death of Samuel Hahnemann it was left to the profession to introduce various drugs. As far as Tuberculinum and its varieties are concerned there are a lot of flaws. As far as its origin and provings are concerned strongly recommend the profession to kindly read in detail the Bibliographic references which are given at the end of this book.

23rd August 1992   **Farokh Jamshed Master**
Vatcha Gandhi Memorial
Bldg. No. 1, Hughes Road,
Bombay-400 007

PREFACE TO SECOND EDITION

After the first edition in 1992, there were two re-prints in 1994 and 1996. This clearly showed that the book was well received by my colleagues. I am happy to inform you that the second edition is now translated into the German language for my German friends.

In preparation of this edition, I have re-written chapters on Portrait of Tuberculinum, Bacillinum and also on Tubercular diathesis and dyscrasias. I hope this edition will be accepted with the same enthusiasm as my other publications.

I am grateful to the following doctors for their help received in the preparation of this edition.

- **Dr. Ameet Panchal**
- **Dr. Piroja Bharucha**
- **Dr. Priya Panchal**
- **Dr. Naini Shah**
- **Dr. Ajay Jain**
- **Dr. Sri Vidya Sreenivasan**
- **Dr. Firuzi Dabu**
- **Dr. Neha Tanna**
- **Dr. Benaifer Mistry**
- **Dr. Shahenaz Khan**

7

ACKNOWLEDGEMENT

I want to express great gratitude and thanks to Dr. Afshan Deshmukh, Dr. Kehkashan Deshmukh, Dr. Diana Minbottiwala, Dr. Zenobia Colabewalla, Dr. Renuka Naik, Dr. Sherbanno Reshamwala, Dr. Zubin Marolia, Dr. Ronak Shah, Dr. Kamal Rustomjee, Dr. Niloufer Bamji, Dr. Devika Pooran, and whose many observations, ideas and long hours of work are represented in these pages.

Without them, this book would still be another idea in the mind of a dreamer.

Dr. S.G. Samant, Dr. K.N. Kasad my senior teachers of Homoeopathic Philosophy, taught me to care for others and supported me in the writing of this book.

Mr. Kuldeep Jain oversaw this project and brought the book to fruition. Mr. Dara Icchaporia as usual designed the cover page so beautifully.

Miss Roda Bandrawala who was a great help.

CONTENTS

CONTENTS

INTRODUCTION

Nosodes are remedies dervied from diseased tissues and secretions containing the specific organism of the disease. The only way to use a nosode is to prove it on the healthy, and note its symptoms, in the recognised way for provings.

One of the commonest nosodes used is Tuberculinum. We employ both the Tuberculous extracts and the anti-tubercular serums in our practice. Let us revise them in detail.

1. Tuberculinum Kochs

Dr. Koch extracted human tubercular bacilli in 1882.

It is a glycerine extract of a pure cultivation of tubercle bacilli (human).

Preparations have been made from Tubercular abscesses derived from the human body, though the infection was probably a bovine strain. (C.E. Wheeler)

It has also been prepared from a drop obtained from a pulmonary tubercular abscess or sputum – prepared and proved by Dr. Swan (186) studies of Homoeopathic

Remedies (Doughlas Gibson). It is a glycerine extract of a pure cultivation of human tubercle bacilli liquid attenuations – M. Bhattacharya & Co's Homoeopathic Pharmacopoeia.

The old Tuberculinum of Koch is specific for pulmonary tuberculosis, as well as a good remedy for suppurations. The new Tuberculinum of Koch is preferred by Trudeau because it has a lesser tendency to cause a febrile reaction.

Features of Tuberculinum Koch :

Weak thin children with flat chest.

Always tired, nevertheless restless, nervous.

Aversion to slightest physical and mental exertion.

Easily exhausted

Tendency to perspiration

Sensitivity to cold and every change of weather

Mentally precocious

Irritable.

Desire for constant change.

Indications:

1. All illness of tubercular genesis, mainly onset of pulmonary T.B. T.B. meningitis (headache, dizziness, tinitus)

2. Erythema nodosum.

3. Ill effects of T.B. vaccination.

4. Rheumatoid arthritis.

5. Otitis media – persistent foul smelling secretion from ear.

6. Neurodermatitis.

7. Chronic eczema on eyelid.

8. Headaches – after school work.

9. Sleep disturbance during second half of night.

10. Rolling of head, waking fearful.

B.C.G.

The vaccine B.C.G. is meant for protecting against Tuberculous infections and is prepared from mycobacterium tuberculosis var hominis bovis. It is constituted by a suspension of microbes coming from the subcultures of the artificially attenuated stock, as described by A. Calmette and Guerin under the name of stock B.C.G.

Indications:-

Student's headache.

Insomnia of students.

Depressive of students.

Depressive Psychoneurosis.

-Chronic hypotension.

-Chronic rhinitis, tonsillitis, etc.

Tuberculinum Bovinum:

Prepared by Kent from the infected lymph glands of cattle and potentised by Boericke and Tafel.

Indications:

1. Catches cold easily.
2. Symptoms constantly changing
3. Love for travel
4. Emaciation.
5. Worse standing
6. Likes refined cuisine, sweets, cold milk, ham, smoked meats, wine.
7. Worse from music.
8. Chronic cystitis.
9. Fear of dogs.
10. Palms of hands – damp.
11. Perspiration only on the nose (characteristic)

Tuberculinum Aviare:

Tuberculinum prepared from bird or chicken liver.

Indications:

1. Incessant tickling cough – acute or chronic.
2. Bronchial pneumonia.
3. Pulmonary affections with profuse expectoration.
4. Influenzal Bronchitis.
5. Itching of palms and ears.
6. Improves appetite if lost.
7. Otitis media – slow onset – difficult hearing.
8. Bronchial ashma – with fever.
9. Restless children
10. Weak children

According to Jose Galard, Aviare is especially indicated when the symptoms are acute and are of such a nature that they may develop into bronchoneumonia. Wheeler prefers it in the exacerbations of chronic pulmonary affections with profuse expectoration.

Tuberculinum of Denys :

It is Denys of Louvain who prepared this product – 1896.

It is made by the French from filtered broth in which tubercular bacilli were grown.

The filtered Bouillon of Denys was a tuberculin prepared after the separation of the microbes by filtration on bougie and concentrated.

According to Calmette it contains a thermolabile toxalbumin which differentiates itself from classical tuberculins. It is used in sudden attacks of depression and weakness with nausea, diarrhoea, vomiting etc.

Serum of marmoreck :

It was in 1903 that marmoreck exposed the encouraging results obtained with this serum. It is obtained from horses vaccinated by the filtrates of young cultures of tubercular bacilli. According to the first observation of Dr. L. Vaunier, Marmoreck may be used in two categories of diseases. The tuberculins and tuberculars.

According to this author the clinical aspects of tuberculins are as follows:

1. Fever without a precise aetiology.
2. Repeated coryza
3. Dental troubles
4. Constipation
5. Cardiac neurosis

All these types may benefit by the use of one or many doses of Marmoreck.

As regards the real tubercular patients, the prescription of the nosode is indicated in tubercular patients having dificient reticulo endothelial reactions, in fibro-caseous forms, in the tuberculosis of bones, tubercular peritonitis and renal tuberculosis.

Tuberculinum Rosebach :

It is made from tubercular bacilli grown symbiotically with dry trycophyton, useful in lupus.

Tuberculinum Residium :

Cultures of tubercular bacilli in Santon medium are heated at 100 c for an hour then filtered. The bacillary mass remaining on the filter paper is washed several times, centrifuged, heated and then decongealed. This is carried out 10 times to cause complete lysis of the bacillary bodies. The Homogenous ground mass thus obtained, is suspended in water and shaken for an hour. It is now centrifuged in suspension of glycerine and filtered. The opalescent liquid thus obtained constitues the residual tuberculinum.

Indication :

1. Fibrositis
2. Rheumatic complaints better motion – sensitivity to weather changes.
3. Finger contractions.
4. Stiffness of forearms – persistent writers cramps.

Bacillinum Testium :

Burnett writes that it is prepared from tuberculous testicles.

Indications :

It acts especially on lower half of the body.

VARIOUS PREPARATIONS OF TUBERCULINS

1. Tuberculinum (Swan and Fincke).
2. Bacillinum (Burnett).
3. Tuberculinum (koch's).
4. Tuberculinum (Koch's Residual).
5. Koch's Lymph.
6. Aviare.
7. Serum of Jousset.
8. Allergme of jousset.
10. Dilute Serum of Marmoreck.
11. Tuberculinum bovinum (Kent).
12. Human Tuberculin of Klebs.

13. Immunising bodies of Spengler.

14. Dialysed Tuberculin.

15. Autogenous products.

16. Vaccine of Bossan.

17. Serum of Movigliano.

18. Pulverised Bacillary emulsion of Hallock.

19. Vaccine of Vaudremer.

20. Chloroformed Tuberculin.

21. Bacilli of Ostermann.

22. Electronic Bacillinum of Whiting.

23. Tuberculinum Porcinus.

24. Bacillinum Testicum.

25. Diluted B.C.G.

26. Sefum of Ferran.

THE SECONDARY SYMPTOMS OF TUBERCULOSIS

MIND

Child of the union of Syphilitic and Psoric dyscrasias presents a picture of the "problem child" slow in comprehension dull, unable to keep a line of thought unsocial – keeps to himself and becomes sullen and morose.

Alternately, cheerfulnes optimism and hopefulness especially in terminal states is a strong indication for tubercular state.

A State of changefulness (May even be hysterical): borne out by a constant urge to travel or for a change of locality.

Fair, intelligent, precocious person with increased sexual desire easily forming intense emotional bonds and consequently many physical and mental symptoms arise from a disappointment in love.

The heightened manifestation of psoric phenomena must be considered to be tubercular in nature; for e.g. restlessness is a psoric trait but when this restlessness is so increased as to drive the patient to disturb others and to make a general nuisance of himself, it is considered to be tubercular.

Patient's mental symptoms are better by the outbreak of an ulcer. Many tubercular states are ameliorated by diarrhoea.

HEAD:

Headaches occurring every Sunday or on rest days, worse ridding in carriage, or due to the least of ordeals, as preparing for emaination; meeting with strangers and entertaining them. Headaches with deathly coldness of hands and feet, with prostration, sadness and general despondency. Headaches with red face and rush of blood to head, or at certain hours of the day, usually in the forenoon; headaches better rest, quiet, sleep, eating.

Headache better nose-bleed. In fact, any symptom better by nosebleed is tubercular. Prosopalgia or persistent headache not easily ameliorated by treatment. Chronic neuralgias fall mainly under sycotic miasm. Tubercular (or syphilitic) headache will often last for days and is very severe, often unendurable, sometimes with sensation of bands about the head.

In the tubercular or syphilitic headaches of children, they strike, knock or pound their heads with their hands or against some object.

OUTER HEAD:

Hair dry like tow, dead like hemp from old rope.

Hair moist, glues together: Moist eruption in hair, better by bathing.

Musty odour from hair like old hay.

Foetid, sour, oily (child).

Crooked, bent, curved or broken eyelashes; imperfect lashes.

THE SCALP :

Pustular eruptions with thick yellowish bland pus.

Offensive discharges from behind and about the ears. Cracks about the ear.

Moist eczematous erruptions about scalp

Scalp is moist, perspiring copiously (Children)

Head large, bulging, often open sutures, soft, cartilaginous (children).

Scalp eruptions moist copious pus formation.

A thick yellow heavy crust is apt to be tubercular or syphilitic in origin.

Matting eruptions

Seborrhoea

Impetigo.

Heat of head worse at night

Aversion to having head uncovered.

EYES AND VISION:

Structural alternations.

Astigmatism and other refractory changes due to malformation. Changes in the lens or in the sclera, choroid, ciliary body and iris.

Processes that change organs and occur as perversions of form and shape or, size (these are also syphilitic)

Photophobia much more marked in Tuberculosis and Syphilis.

Dreads artificial light more than sunlight.

Disturbance in the glandular structures or in the lach-, rymal apparatus (also in Syphilis). Pustular diseases as found in many cases of granular lids. Dacryocystitis, trachoma.

Ulcerations and specific inflammation: ciliary blepharitis acute or chronic (also in Syphilis), scaly red lids, angry looking.

Thick copious pus formation or discharges especially if greenish or yellowish-green, are .distinctly tubercular or sycotic.

Ciliary neuralgia.

Rheumatic eye troubles like rheumatic iritis, Reiter's syndrome, and Sjorgen's syndrom. Generally better by hot applications. Phlyctenular conjunctivitis-worse night, after sunset.

Styes on eyes.

A chronic dilatation of the pupil in children or women. When these patients are affected with exanthematous fevers of any form there is a strong tendency to inflammatory stasis of the eye, and serious eye troubles are apt to follow.

Lachrymal fistula.

Glaucoma: inflammation of angle of filtration

Oculomotor paralysis.

EAR AND HEARING:

All organic ear troubles especially affecting the middle ear.

Suppurative process and destruction of the ossicles of the ears.

Ears are often a safety valve in tubercular children. Abscesses relieve quite severe meningeal difficulties. They show up frequently in measles, scarlet fever, etc. Here the tubercular element comes readily to the surface in the form of suppuration of the middle ear. More frequently aroused by fever.

Peculiar, carrion-like odour from these aural abscesses are very characteristic.

Often discharges cheesy or curdled.

Exanthemata – ears.

If free from ear troubles these children invariably suffer from throat affections, especially tonsillitis. They appear well in the day time and free from pain but at night their sufferings begin, and they often scream with earache. They may begin as early as the first year and go on until puberty. The least exposure to cold or slightest draft brings on an attack. Occasionally we have prolonged febrile attacks with great suffering and suddenly better by the breaking of an abscess. Quite often their general health is better even when the ear is discharging copiously, this tubercular, four-smelling pus.

Ears look pale, often cold, and in some cases translucent almost with the blood vessels enlarged, bluish in colour or bright red. (also in Syphilis)

Eczematous eruptions about the ears and especially the humid eruptions, pustules, fissures and incrustations behind the ear.

NOSE AND SMELL:

Nose haemorrhages are profuse, bright red difficult to arrest and are better by cold applications. Over heating & over exercise will often bring them on.

The tubercular child will have a haemorrhage from the nose on the slightest provocation – blowing the nose, a slight blow, or washing the face, will produce it in some people.

Headache, vertigo and congestion to the brain and head are often ameliorated by nose-bleeds.

In worst form of hay fever where there is much sneezing with much local troubles it often depends on the tubercular taint with an acquired latent sycosis.

Discharge soon becomes thick, purulent and sometimes bloody.

Rush of blood to surface inducing great heat.

Catarrhal discharge is thick, usually yellow an of the odour of old cheese or sulphate of hydrogen and is constantly dropping down the throat.

FACE:

Eyes sunken with blue rings.

Circumscribed red spot on cheeks, usually appearing in the afternoon or evening.

Flushes of heat to face, head and chest.

Red lips where blood is almost ready to ooze out.

Reddish millet sized papules on nose, cheeks, chin and ulcers in corners of mouth.

Deep fissures in lips. Hectic flushes on nose, cheeks, chin and ulcers in corners of mouth. Acne Rosacea.

Deep fisures in lips. Hectic flushes in fever. In tubercular fever face is pale or with circumscribed red spots on cheeks.

Paleness of face on rising and even after eating. One cheek red, the other pale; one cheek hot, the other cold.

Tubercular face is round, skin fair, smooth and clear, with that waxy smoothness of complexion; eyes bright and sparkling, eyebrows and eyelashes soft, glossy, long and silken, thin lips.

We have the high cheek bones, and thick lips, In some cases the skin of the face is rough, voice coarse, deep, often hollow, eyelids red, inflammed, scaly, crusty lashes, broken, stubby, irregularly curved and imperfect. In these case the syphilitic or tubercular element predominates in latent form.

The face and head is often seen to be in the shape of a pyramid, with apex at the chin. The nose may be well shaped, the features sharp, eyes usually bright and sparkling, nostrils small, openings narrow and the least obstruction in the nose induces them to breathe through the mouth, which causes in imperfect expansion and filling of the lungs.

We may not see the flashes of heat or circulatory expressions we see in the other expressions of the tubercular face; indeed the face looks fairly well even in the last stages of disease, when other parts of the body become emaciated and show marked signs of the disease.

With hopefulness and cheerfulness.

Suppurating pustular – deep pitted disfigured.

MOUTH:

True ulcers. Painful, undermined edges.

Swelling and induration of glands and such pathological changes as we see taking place in the teeth or dental arches are of a syphilitic or tubercular diathesis. Dental arches or teeth malformed.

Haemorrhage of mouth, excessive bleeding of gums (unless Syphilis is actually present)- often they will bleed at slightest touch. Gums recede from teeth or they are soft and spongy. The dental arch is imperfect, irregular, or teeth are imperfect in form, club-shaped, or they come in an irregular order, often a decaying or becoming carious before they are entirely through the gums they appear often with much pain and suffering, accompanied with constitutional disturbances, often of a marked degree, such as diarrhoea, dysentery, spasms, convulsion, febrile states, abscesses of the middle ear, disturbance of digestion, meningeal congestions, and meningeal inflammations. These children cannot endure extremes of heat and cold. Worse dentition during. Pharyngeal abscess, chronic tubercular cervical spine Recurrent tonsillitis with cervical glands with suppuration.

Pharyngitis following tonsillectomy.

TASTE:

Putrid or taste of blood or pus. Expectoration of pus that tastes sweet. Salty taste or a rotten-egg taste.

Taste of blood; it may not come during menstrual period but is present frequently in the morning.

All metallic tastes make us think of tubercular or a syphilitic element.

DESIRES AND AVERSION:

Extreme: like hot or cold things.

Long for indigestible things-chalk, lime, slate, pencils, etc.

If the system is not assimilating a certain thing they will crave it (and it is the peculiarity of tubercular patients. H. Choudhary); this is seen more in young girls, in children and in pregnant women. They are craves for peculiar things; salt, and will eat it alone from the dish. They eat more salt than all the family put together. Long for stimulants, beer, wines or hot aromatic things.

Craves potatoes and meat, salt, salty fish, cold.

Craving for unnatural things to eat, with desire for narcotics such as tea, coffee, tobacco and any other stimulants, have often their origin in psoric or tubercular Miasm.

Aversion to fats and meat.

Aggravation from starchy foods.

HUNGER:

Faint if hunger is not satisfied or extreme hunger with all gone, weak, empty feelings in the stomach (but with psoric origin).

They sometimes have constant hunger and eat beyond their capacity to digest or they have no appetite in the morning but hunger for other meals.

Great desire for certain thing but when he receives them he does not want them; in fact they are repugnant to him. (We see this perhaps more in children than in adults).

Capricious.

Hunger headaches.

Ravenous appetite, yet emaciates.

STOMACH:

Weak, "all-gone" sensation.

Crave meat.

Crave meat, many reject the fat.

Thrive better on fats and fat foods; also require much salt. Starches are not easily digested by them.

Desires salty fish.

Desires cold things to eat and drink.

Hiatus hernia.

Bleedings.

ABDOMEN:

Peritoneal inflammation.

Patients easily chilled about the abdomen causing colic, diarrhoea or dysentery and may severe bowel troubles follow.

We often find the worst forms of constipation or inactivity of the bowels in psoric or tubercular patients.

You can often feel the beating of the abdominal aorta through the abdominal wall.

In children we find ulceration of umbilicus with yellowish discharge, which smells offensive, carrion-like.

In menstrual difficulties we may find reflex pains, spasmodic symptoms and bearing down sensation, especially in tubercular patients. Skin is pale with an underlying bluish tint showing the venous stagnation.

Hernia-seldom found outside the tubercular organism.

Usually found in flabby, soft-muscled people. Hernia is due to this lack of tone in the muscled system through out the whole abdominal region. The shape of the Tuberculinum abdomen is saucer-shaped or as a large plate turned bottom side up.

Skin-pale with underlying bluish tint, abdominal Hodgkins.

BOWEL AND INTESTINAL TRACT :

Abdomen very sensitive to cold esp. in infants.

Morning aggravation in bowel troubles. Still more sensitive to cold, which aggravates.

In bowel difficulties, gone empty feeling in the abdominal region; sometimes it is a great weakness after stool, felt only in the region of the abdomen (also in psoric cases).

General exhaustion or loss of strength a feeling as if all vitality is leaving the patient at each evacuation of the bowels. Debilitating diarrhoea, debilitating cholera infantum.

True syphilitic or tubercular patients are worse at night; they are driven out of bed by their diarrhoeas, sometimes this is accompanied with profuse warm or cold perspiration which is very exhausting and debilitating.

It is characteristic of these tubercular children suffering from bowel troubles to develop a sudden brain stasis, or brain metastasis. Sometimes the tubercular manifestations in the brain alternate with a bowel difficulty.

Ver.alb., Ars., Camph, and Cup.met diarrhoea and dysenteries are characteristic in tubercular patients. They look well today, have a sudden attack of dysentery and are dead within 48 hours.

Podo has painless, copious, yellowish and very offensive stool, worse at night and morning and worse from milk. A Tubercular child cannot use cow's milk in any from. Least exposure to cold brings on diarrhoea in tubercular children.

On beginning or eruption of the first teeth, diarrhoea starts in tubercular babies; plus at this stage loss of power to assimilate bone-making material in food.

Crot.tig.: stool of tubercular children is strongly trained with Sycosis.

Sang., Phos., Kali.c, Tuber and Stan. are typical of the tubercular discharges.

Sometimes in tubercular children stools are ashy or grey in colour showing lack of bile matter.

Bloody stools.

Child smells musty-mouldy.

In severe cases of bowel trouble child is fretful, peevish and whiny, does not want to be touched or looked at; prostration after stools marked.

They are worse milk, potatoes, meat and worse motion.

Before stool there is often vomiting and retching

Diarrhoea ameliorates. Bleeding piles. Actinomycosis.

Stool with much slimy mucus or much blood passes after stool.

T.B. abdomen.

T.B. peritonitis.

T.B. enteritis.

Tabes mesenterica.

Crohn's disease.

Intestinal infestations (helminths).

Pin worms or intestinal worms are found more plentiful in children with tubercular taint.

Rectal diseases (fistula as concomitant) alternating with heart chest or lung troubles, especially of asthma and respiratory difficulties; e.g. haemorrhoids if operated on or suppressed are followed by lung difficulties or asthma and not infrequently by heart troubles.

Haemorrhage from rectum. Prolapsus of rectum in young children. The bowel difficulties are frequently accompanied with febrile states, delirium, gastric disturbances, vomiting, purging with exhaustive purging stools. Cancerous affections, malignant growths and such diseases have as a rule all the miasms present-especially the Sycotic and Tubercular combined.

Psora can never be left out of malignancies no matter what other element may combine with it; it fathers them all.

Stricture rectum (including lymphogranuloma venereum) Sinuses, fistulae and fistulous pockets (Multiple sinuses inguinal buboes with suppuration). Pruritus ani-diabetic.

URINARY ORGANS

Anxiety and much loss of strength after urination. T.B. urinary tract.

In tubercular diathesis, especially in nervous or neurotic patients. Urine is pale, colourless and copious with very little solids present.

Diabetic patients have strong tubercular diathesis.

Bright's disease.

Urine offensive and easily decomposed, odour musty, like old hay or foul smelling-even carrion-like.

In tubercular children urine may be involuntary at night as soon as they fall asleep. Also copious. This is why Calc. cures so many as the tubercular Miasm is tackled.

Idiopathic hydrocoele.

Prostatic trouble in cases where we have constant loss of the prostatic or seminal fluid, consumption sometimes develops.

These patients live in gloom with depressed spirits, gloomy forebodings, poor digestion, loss of energy, want of memory. Livid or ashy complexion, appetite often voracious as system calls for more food than it can properly take care of, when finally gastric derangements follow, until the organism fails to perform any function in a proper manner.

In rectum we find many conditions of tubercular origin as strictures, fistulae, sinuses and pockets.

SEXUAL SPHERE:

Reflex symptoms, bearing down sensations.

Many psyco-sexual perversions-these may be even worse in the tubercular patient.

Menstruation exhaustive and often prolonged and copious flow. Haemorrhage bright red, sometimes accompanied with vertigo, faintness, and with pallor, worse by rising from recumbent position. Frequently they are too soon, appearing every 2 to 3 weeks; they may or may not be painful but are always exhausting; Feels badly a week before.

Suffering in many ways with headaches, backaches, gastric disturbances, neuralgias, etc. Occasionally menses appear with diarrhoea, with epistaxis, with febrile states, optical illusions roaring in the ears, sensitiveness to noise, loss of appetite, abnormal pains, nausea and bitter vomiting.

After the flow patient looks pale with dark rings or circles about eyes; or hollow eyed with a worn, exhausted look. Hysterical symptoms often arise, of any form of degree in severity and often they are most difficult to treat.

Flow is often pale, watery and long lasting, as seen in Calc. C, Ferrum, etc.

Extremities are usually cold and often menstrual flow will induce general anaemia in young women from 17 to 21 years of age. They become chlorotic.

Often complexion becomes pale, assuming yellowish or ashen hue, accompanied by starchy or watery leucorrhoea, palpitation of the heart, faintness and loss of vitality; general weakness, flushing in the face, vertigo, ringing in the ears, hoarseness, dry tickling spasmodic cough and finally a true tubercular condition develops. Often they are very sad, gloomy anxious, full of fanciful notion, forebodings with much fear extreme sensitiveness, nervous irritability and inclination to weep. Menses bright red, or light coloured and watery.

We sometimes see nausea and vomiting, extreme purging of the bowels, with diarrhoea or dysentery, cold sweat on the forehead, but flow is seldom. If ever clotted; being usually fluid, profuse, light red, watery, offensive and not infrequently it has the odour of fresh blood.

Leucorrhoea usually purulent but may be watery mucus.

Patient often debilitated and worse before flow or immediately after it begins.

Deep, thick yellow or yellowish green. Sometimes lumpy, thick albuminous or purulent.

Smelling musty. Cervical erosions.

Sterility.

Fecundity.

Nocturnal emissions.

Retroversion, retroflexions, and malpositions of uterus, prolapse.

In marked cases of this diathesis uterus is retroverted or retroflexed and many sufferings date from puberty.

Labour and childbirth are often difficult, severe, prolonged and exhausting and many are unable to nurse their children.

Sexual perversions
Lascivious.

UPPER AND LOWER EXTREMITIES:

Neuralgic pains either psoric or tubercular usually better by quiet rest and warmth. Often worse motion and better rest and warmth.

Tubercular joint troubles, increase in osseous tissue, nodular growth similar to syphilis. Bones are soft, rickety and curved. Syphilitic element feet become deformed because legs cannot take weight of body.

The periosteal difficulties are due to periosteal inflammations or tertiary or tubercular changes in the bones themselves.

The tubercular and syphilitic bone and periosteal pains are very similar both as to their character and times of aggravation. T.B. spine (Pott's Disease).

Cold abscess, psoas abscess.

Caries of bone with suppuration leading to sinuses and fistulae.

Tubercular tenosynovitis.

Varicose veins.

In nails we may have inflammatory changes due to Syphilis and Tuberculosis. We have in both, true onychosis though not of such specific character in the tubercular process as in tertiary Syphilis.

Paronychia is tubercular as met with in pale-skinned, anaemic tubercular subjects. Pustules form often on lower extremities or about fingers or hands. Felons. Soft easily tearing nails.

The nails of these patients are brittle, break of split easily, often hang-nails.

Nails thin as paper, bend easily and are sometimes spoon shaped; the natural convexity is reversed.

Spotted nails, or show white specks-sometimes anterior edges are serrated or slightly scalloped. Often nails drop off and grow again.

Periosteal inflammation commonly known as felons or periphalangeal cellulitis.

Fingers are long and do not-taper gradually but are blunt or clubshaped at 'extremities". This long fingered individual with the lengths so irregularly arranged is characteristic. Often the hand is thin, soft and flabby and easily compressed.

The same, regarding feet; coldness of hands and feet is very marked but the patient is not always conscious of it.

Hang-nails.

We see such types in remedies such as Calc. C. Bar.C., Bar.Iod. Iodine and Silicea.

General tissue atonia.

Prolapses.

Displacements.

Herniations – internal and external.

Dislocations.

Sprains.

Ankel turning.

Heat and cold aggravates.

Warm air very annoying, cannot endure much cold neither can they endure much heat.

Chilblains are based on all the miasms-we have the tubercular taint, with a sycotic element as basis. That is why they prove to be dreadful disease producing agent when suppressed by local measures- Madura foot.

Boils they may depend on both psoric and tubercular influences.

Boils with such suppuration.

Paralytic disease, oedematous swellings, anasarca are Sycotic, Syphilitic & Tubercular. General muscular weakness and loss of power in ankles.

Clumsy-awkward, lack of co-ordination-they are always falling. They drop things. They tire easily when walking and especially when climbing.

This patient is short-winded, climbing stairs tires out the patient.

White swellings of joints or idiopathic synovitis even rheumatic forms have this tubercular element very marked.

Drop wrist, weakness or loss of power in tendons about joint. In children and young people, ligaments about joints easily sprained, ankles turn-easily from the slightest mis-step, wrists show the same weakness, playing the piano or operating a typewriter causes swelling, soreness or pain in wrist joints. Lack energy as well as strength.

Weakness of the ankle joints is a sure indication of the presence of a Syphilitic taint in combination with the Psoric stigma.

Weakness of ankles.

Leprosy.

THE SKIN:

Skin affections with glandular involvement will necessarily have the syphilitic or tubercular element to conform with glandular involvement.

In varicose veins the tubercular taint predominates, and it is in these patients that we see the varicose ulcers, the last skin lesion to make its appearance in a case of ancient or hereditary syphilis that has already become, and now is largely tubercular.

In ecchymosis or any form of purpura there is a tubercular basis.

Impetigo, leprosy.

Eczema-Pustular – especially about ears with cracks.

Herpes zoster.

Urticaria.

Hyperhidrosis and Bromhidrosis

Anhydrosis.

Abscess and ulcers – painful with undermined edges.

Freckles.

Fine, smooth, clear skin.

Goose flesh, (Nat.m., Hep and Sil.)

Abscess and ulcerations after injuries.

Bee and bugs affect these patients badly.

Gangrene.

The patients often have benign or malignant tumours.

In tubercular and syphilitic patients we see much scarring and increase in cicatrical tissue.

Leprosy.

In the lymphatic temperament we see the malignancies, we find here rich soil for gonorrhoea and Syphilis. In tubercular patients we have much difficulty in eradicating acquired syphilis or gonorrhoea.

Gonorrhoea runs to gleety discharge and strictures, pockets and metastasis form, or we have metastasis to ovaries, broad ligaments, tubes, uterus, rectum and all such complications. It is the tubercular Diathesis that complicates all our skin disease and makes them so difficult to remove.

Supress any or of ringworm and there often follows Tubercular diseases (Burnett) Sycosis on a Tubercular base.

Vaccination leading to encephalitis, epilepsy suppuration.

All skin diseases are triple miasmatic.

CHEST, HEART & LUNGS :

Phthisis – Pulmonalis, Tuberculosis, consumption.

The curves and lines of chest are imperfect, the chest is often narrow, lacking not only width laterally, but depth anterior posteriorly, the subclavicular spaces are hollow or certain areas sunken or depressed, quite often one lung is larger than the other, or the action of one is accelerated and the other lessened; one side is fuller than the other, showing a better development and a greater respiratory area, often the expansive power of the lung is greatly limited and the amount of residual air lessened.

Breathing is not so full and resonant, although there may be impediment or obstruction in the air cells of passages. Shoulders are rounded, inclined forward infringing on the chest and the free lung action. Poor breathers, they have no desire to take a full respiration, seldom do we find them breathing diaphragmatically, thus the lung never comes to its fullest expansion and the air cells are not brought into use and simply become diseased from lack of that life-giving oxygen they should received. From the lack of work they atrophy and become useless, the least obstruction glues them together and destroys their office.

Faulty nutrition.

Afraid of cold air which aggravates.

Worse on least exposure to cold.

Voice hoarse, deep with bass-like chest tones, slightly sore at times, a rawness and a croak-like sound develop in voice; constant desire to hawk or clear throat of a viscid, scantly mucus, (sore throats of Hep and Phos) Tracheitis.

Cough deep-prolonged, worse morning and when patient first lies down in evening. Expectoration purulent, or mucopurulent and in advanced cases, greenish yellow, often offensive and usually sweetish to taste, or salty (dependable indications of the combined psoric and syphilitic taints sometimes it smells musty or offensive.

In these cases there is gradual failing away of the flesh, rush of blood to the chest and face.

41

The dyspnoea is often painful in psoric or tubercular patients.

The dropsies or the anasarcas of the psoric or tubercular patients are always greater than sycotic they smother or drown the patient before death takes place may be bloody or followed by haemorrhage. Cough deep ringing, hollow, no expectoration or none to speak of.

Cough can be dry and tight and induce headache, or whole body shaken by paroxysms.

EXPECTORATION

The expectoration is usually greenish or yellow, thick and viscid, often easily discharged and with an offensive odour.

HEART

A rush of blood to the chest and face, especially in the young.

Heart troubles are accompanied with fainting, temporary loss of vision, ringing in the ears, pallor and great weakness, worse sitting up and usually better by lying down.

Cannot climb mountains as disturbed circulation affects the brain and they become dizzy and faint, often fainting away when they get to a rarified atmosphere. Brain becomes anaemic at a high altitude.

Sense of great exhaustion, easily made tired, never seems to get rested, tired at night, tired even after sleep, as the day advances they become better or as the sun ascends their strength revives a little, as it descends, they lose it again.

There is a sense of constriction or oppression or tightness in the region of the heart.

There are palpitations which occur more in the evening after eating. Palpitations are often accompanied with pain in the back and vertigo. Palpitations are worse during cough, when the patient takes a deep breath and when lying on the side.

There is a sensation as if the heart were swinging by a thread.

These patients are often worse in the night, which they dread and they long for morning.

Look out for patients with the nightly aggravation, no matter what the pathology may be.

The non-resistance of the tissues, the slightest bruise suppurates the strong tendency is to pustules the same may be said of the expectoration of the lungs-its pus-like nature and copiousness.

Pneumoconiosis;

Boeck's Sarcoidosis.

Pneumonia

Hodgkin's – mediastinum

Chronic Mycosis

A PORTRAIT OF TUBERCULINUM

PHYSICAL MAKE-UP

Emaciation, marasmus.

Slender built.

Stoop-shouldered.

Tall, slim, narrow-chested. Caved-in chest.

Thin or oval face frame.

Hair soft and silky. Covered with fine hair all over.

Eye lashes long.

Fine textured skin.

CLINICAL NOTES:

Relapsing, recurring states.

Repeated exacerbations of local symptoms.

For example.

- Pretubercular conditions.
- Intermittent fevers.
- Low grade recurring fevers.
- Chronic diarrhoeas.
- Chronic headaches.
- Recurring catarrhal conditions.

- Patients who have been treated with antibiotics and cortisone for mild illnesses.
- Chronic tonsillitis.
- Chronic otitis media.
- Chronic cases of enuresis.
- Chronic cases of ringworm.
- People with any chronic illness, having a tubercular constitution who respond marginally to the seemingly indicated remedies require **TUBERCULINUM.**

THE TUBERCULAR "TYPE"

1. Febrile without apparent reason.
2. Persons subject to continuous colds.
3. Frequent dental case.
4. Constipated individuals.
5. Cardiac patients especially functional heart disease.
6. Pulmonary T.B.
7. Fatigue.
8. Family H/O T.B.
9. Fear of dogs and cats.
10. Desires-smoked meat, sweets, bread, bacon, milk.
11. Strong desire for OPEN AIR.
12. Desire for TRAVEL.
13. > cold weather
14. > in the mountains.

15. < motion (in severe pains in joints).
16. Emaciation with great appetite.
17. Flushing.
18. Alopecia of beard, tinea barbae.

MENTAL SYMPTOMS INCLUDING MENTAL STATES

1 RESTLESSNESS : (Physical as well as mental)
Cannot tolerate standing still or any fixed position.
> walking fast
Tuberculinum patients select jobs involving movement and travel eg.,

- Postman.
- Air hostess.
- Broker.
- Deliver man.
- Salesman.
- Medical representative.

A young adolescent roams the city during his free time.

A restless housewife repeatedly goes to the Bazaar on the slightest pretext.

II. MENTAL

Intellectual desultoriness.
Capriciousness.
Dissatisfaction.

It can be said of Tuberculinum patients that their "INTEREST IS A MILE WIDE AND AN INCH DEEP" Eg.,

- Cannot complete a novel
- Turns pages of magazines or newspaper 100 quickly.

EASILY DISTRACTED

Can concentrate better when on the move or when outdoors. Eg.,

- Travelling on a trains, aeroplane, etc.
- Waiting in a queue at the bus stop.

Common expressions of changeability, as observed in practice: Change of :-

- Schools, colleges.
- Career.
- Jobs on the slightest pretext.
- Hobbies.
- Physician.
- Friends.
- Profession.
- Homes, i.e., will stay for a few days with one relative then with another.

III. DESIRE TO TRAVEL AND DISCOVER- A true cosmopolitan

- Excitedly and fancifully anticipates every outing or journey.
- Sense of adventure
- Sensation that life is too short so must be lived to the hilt.

Illustration :- from life situation observed in my practice.

If a patient is incapable of travelling physically, he has fantasies of travel. He reads the National Geographic Magazine or sees a move which is picturised on outdoor locales or reads travel brochures or watches T.V. programmes on travelling and often they like to work for an Airline company, Merchant Navy or Travel Agencies for the opportunities it offers them to visit new places.

IV. ALTERNATION OF MOODS

There are frequent emotional upheavals. The following moods are usually seen:-

- Need for support.
- Inactivity.
- Melancholy.
- Violence.
- Child craves attention.
- Wants independance.
- Restlessness.

- Exhilaration.
- Tenderness.
- Desires to be left alone.

V. AESTHETIC INCLINATION

It can be derived from
- Sensitivity to music heightened inspiration
- Increased spirituality
- Creativity

Usually Tuberculinum patients can play various musical instruments. They frequently visit art galleries, keep antiques in their house, have hobbies like painting, etc.

VI. HEIGHTENED SEXUAL DESIRE

The following points justify the feelings-
- Falling easily and deeply in love
- Easy liberation of romantic feelings for the opposite sex. An ardent, seductive personality with heightened sexual desire.
- Keen interest in sexual matters.
  Eg., watching triple "X" movies.
  Sex magazines, visiting play shops.

VII. HOPEFUL

This is a very strong emotional factor that I have observed, especially in terminally ill patients. Even chronic patients have a strong capacity for hope they strongly believe that they will achieve their desire.

VIII. EMOTIONAL TURMOIL

- Civilised.
- Artistic.
- Cultured CONFLICT.
- Decent.
- Sober.
- Longing for security.

- Excitement.
- Adventurous.
- Emotional freedom.
- Heightened sexual passion.

This conflict occur largely at the subconscious level and, when thwarted, is expressed in tantrums at the slightest provocation.

Melancholy, restlessness and alternating moods are other features of the Tuberculinum personality.

TUBERCULINUM CHILD

I Would describe the Tuberculinum child by using two words:
1. DISSATISFIED
2. DESTRUCTIVE

DISSATISFIED:

The child can never be satisfied by anything.

Easily changing moods.

The child is extremely capricious.

Rejects things when offered.

Whines and complains with every little ailment.

Trifles irritate.

This leads to fits of violent temper characterised by:

1.Wants to throw things.

2.Wants to fight.

3.Throws things at anyone even without a cause.

Just when the parents are about to go out the child will throw an ugly tantrum just to spoil their plans

DESTRUCTIVE:

This projects the destructive tendency of Tuberculinum. The child will do exactly what he has been told not to do.

There is a marked fear of animals, especially cats and dogs.

On seeing the animal, the child will cross to the other side of the road.

The child will even refuse to visit a relative who has a dog in his house.

At night the child awakens with a scream on account of nightmares.

At home or at school, he is extremely restless-cannot sit in one place.

Cannot concentrate on one subject for a long time.

The following are the rubrics which depict the Tuberculinum mind:

Abusive.

Break things, desire to.

Cursing.

Destructiveness.

Excitement, excitable.

Fear of dogs.

Moods changeable, variable.

Shrieking.

Typically, the child is a union of syphilitic and psoric dyscrasias presenting to the physician as a problem child.

OUTLINE OF TUBERCULINUM CHILD

Mental/Emotional Characteristics

1. Retardation and slowness
2. Difficulty in comprehension
    (a) Poor concentration
        (i) Physically tires them.
        (ii) Makes them ill.
    (b) Averse to mental activity, will not do homework.
    (c) Memory weakness, must read and reread.
3. Often accompany physical birth anomalies.
4. Dullness may occur
    (a) After illness
    (b) Even in bright children
5. Fears
    (a) Strangers.
    (b) New situations.
    (c) Like Baryta carbonica.

B. Restlessness

1. Intense energy
   a. All day long.
   b. Still energetic at night : restless in sleep
      (i)   Grind teeth.
      (ii) Toss about in bed.
   c. Like to leave the home, go with the parents on errands.
2. May lead to hyperactivity.
   a. Love to run, spin and shout.
   b. Strike others.
   c. Aggravated by eating dairy products.
3. Restlessness in the doctor's office.
   a. Play with many toys.
   b. Bounce on the couch.
   c. Move around.
      (i)   From one object to another.
      (ii) From one chair to another.

C. Irritability

1. Can be born irritable.
2. Especially worse upon awakening.
3. May be continuous or intermittent.
4. Become violent with anger.
   (a) hitting or biting others.
   (b) Throwing fits, striking the head on the ground.
5. May be more mildly irritable: peevish.

D. Contrariness

1. Say or do the opposite of what others wish.
2. May refuse to take the remedy.

E. Destruction and violence

1. Self-destructive : strike themselves, especially on the head.
2. Towards others.

    (a) Hit them: "slaphappy".

    (b) threaten parents in the interview.

3. May be episodic with apologies afterward.
4. Love to sit and cut paper with scissors.
5. Violent towards pets.

F. Selfishness: uncaring

1. About others

    (a) Their persons.

    (b) Their property.

    (c) Their plans.

2. Enjoy ruining all of the above.

G. Teasing, impish character in some

H. Fears

1. Animals.

    (a) Dogs.

    (b) Cats.

2. Being alone.

3. new situations.

I. Sleep

1. Restless.

   (a) While falling asleep.

   (b) During sleep.

2. Sleep very deeply, cannot be awakened easily.

3. Nocturnal enuresis.

4. Almost all will grind their teeth.

5. Night sweats.

6. Sleep positions

   (a) Knee-to-chest.

   (b) On the back with the hands above the head.

7. Very irritable upon awakening.

HEAD:

Morning headaches < sun rise.

> sun set.

Headaches with bilious attacks, nausea and vomiting.

Headache < riding in a carriage.

> preparation for examination.

> quiet sleep.

> rest.

> eating.

> nose bleed.

SCALP:

Hair dry, lusterless, tangles easily, breaks and splits.

Hair becomes white in spots or in streaks.

Hair falls out after abdominal or chest diseases or parturition.

Moist eruptions in the hair, with crust formation.

Offensive odour from head (mousy)

Aversion to having head uncovered.

EYES AND VISION:

Astigmatism and other marked refractory changes due to malformation.

Dreads artificial light.

Ulcerations and specific inflammations with thick copious pus discharges, especially yellowish or yellowish green in colour.

Ciliary neuralgias < night.

> hot application.

Styes.

Glaucoma.

Lachrymal fistula

EARS:

Suppurative process and destruction of the ossicles of the ear.

Persistent offensive otorrhoea

Perforation of tympanum with ragged edges.

NOSE:

Crops of small boils, very painful, successively appear in nose, green fetid pus.

Sweat on the nose.

Colds, end in diarrhoea.

FACE:

Old, oedematous, pale.

Aching in malar bones.

MOUTH:

Feeling as if the teeth were all jammed together and too many for his mouth.

Teeth sensitive to air.

Delayed dentition.

Dryness, stickiness.

Black blisters on lips.

THROAT:

Hawks mucus after eating.

Adenoids.

Dryness of the posterior nares.

Enlarged tonsils.

DESIRES AND AVERSION:

- Craves:

alcoholic drinks.

bacon.
bananas.
butter.
delicacies.
fat.
ham, desires fat.
ice cream.
Meat.
Meat, smoked.
milk.
milk, cold.
pork.
potatoes.
pungent.
refreshing things.
salami.
salt.
smoked food.
spices.
sweets.
warm drinks.
- Aversion to:
food.
meat
milk
cold milk
sweets
wine

- Aggravations:
Coffee.
Warm food.

STOMACH:

All gone hungry sensation which drives one to eat.

ABDOMEN:

Early morning sudden diarrhoea. Stools, brown, watery, discharged with much force.

Tabes mesenteric.

Diarrhoea of children running for weeks, with wasting, exhaustion and bluish pallor.

Tearing in recutm on coughing.

Inguinal glands indurated and visible. Drum belly. Chronic diarrhoea with excessive sweat.

Constipation-stools large and hard, then diarrhoea.

Spleen region bulging out, stitching pain in sides after running.

RESPIRATORY SYSTEM:

Sensation of suffocation, even with plenty of fresh air, longs for cold air.

Hoarseness > talking

Cough-dry, hard, more during sleep, > dyspnoea; with chill and red face> evening; >raising arms; mucus rattle in chest; without expectoration.

Hoarseness talking.

Sore spot in chest.

Asthma. Pneumonia after influenza.

Profuse expectoration. Thick yellow or yellow green sputum.

CARDIO VASCULAR SYSTEM:

Heaviness and pressure over the heart.

Palpitation, on taking deep breath after evening meal.

URINARY SYSTEM:

Must strain at stool to pass water.

Bedwetting.

Sticky urinary sediment.

NECK AND BACK:

Tension in nape.

Pain in back, with palpitation. Chill between shoulders or up the back.

SEXUAL SPHERE:

Female – menses soon after child birth, too early, too profuse, too longlasting.

Dysmenorrhoea-pain increases with the flow.

Mammary tumours-benign.

Amenorrhoea.

Retraction of nipples.

Severe pain in breast at the beginning of menses.

EXTREMITIES:

Hands and arms feel lame, unable to write or raise a cup or a glass.

Fingertips brown.

Sensation of fatigue in limbs.

Cold feet in bed.

Limbs feel weak or as if paralysed, aggravated dinner.

Pains in ulnar nerve.

SKIN:

Dry, harsh, sensitive, easily tanned, itching in cool air. Branny scales.

Psoriasis.

Chronic eczema.

Itching changes places on rubbing.

SLEEP:

Restless at night and screams in sleep.

Shuddering sensation on falling to asleep.

Awakes in horror.

Dreams vivid, of shame, frightful.

FEVER:

Chilly, when beginning to sleep, yet wants fresh air.

Heat on cheek of affected side, in spots.

Flushes of heat < eating.

Burning in genitals.

Sweat-easy, cold, clammy, on upper parts, on hand<
coughing, stains yellow.

Wants covers in all stages of fever.

THE MOTHER'S STATE DURING PREG-NANCY:

It may be a first pregnancy or a pregnancy after a long time, or a precious pregnancy. This leads to a lot of excitement and also anticipation.

- *Ailments from, anticipation, foreboding, presentiment.*
- *Ailments from, excitement, general symptoms from.*

It could also be the case of a working woman, who, because of her socio-economic conditions is not able to take enough rest and hence has to do tremendous amount of mental and physical work. It could also be useful for mothers who are appearing for exams.

- *Ailments from, work mental.*

    There may also be an impending threat which a woman may face about her family.

- *Delusions, people, behind him, someone is*
- *Fear, evil, of, family, impending on his.*
- *Fear, happen, something will, family, to or to him.*

Even though there is no direct abuse, but in my Tuberculinum series, I have witnessed many abuses against the woman during her pregnancy.

63

During the pregnancy, some common dreams encountered are:

- *Dreams, animals, dogs, black.*

  Snakes.

  Fire.

  Prude being.

  Robbers.

  Shameful.

If we try to interpret these dreams, we find that these dreams have a lot to do with "expressing one's inner feelings".

Dreams of dogs—This is an easy expression of our own aspects like aggression, sexuality, friendship; and expression of easy flowing natural feelings.

Dreams of snakes—Snakes depict the life process. The snake actually depicts the force behind a person's purposiveness and movement.

Dreams of fire—fire stands for expression of passion, sexuality, anger, desire, resentment and frustration.

Dreams of robbers — Indicates fears or difficult emotions arising from the unconscious, neglected parts of oneself, which if met with can lead to self-improvement.

Also, it is essential, many times there is a family history of tuberculosis in either parent.

The state of mental faculties will often be the first clue that the child needs tuberculinum.

Children born with mental handicaps like

— Mild learning difficulties.

— Mental retardation.

— Congenital malformations.

eg: Microcephaly.

pectus excavatum.

simian creases on the palms.

oddly shaped fingers.

Enormous variety of chromosomal disorders preponderance to midline anomalies.

During the development of the foetus, more specifically during the earlier embryonic period, there is a stage in which the flat cells that make up the embryo, begin to round off and encapsulate to form a tube. It is as if there is a breakdown at the developmental landmarks causing any of a number of problems including hydrocoele, umbilical hernia and cleft palate, childrens' skulls appear oddly shapen, as if one of the many sutures closed off prematurely. Most of the deformities involve problems with bone and cartilage developments.

{D/D Baryta Carb (fear of new situations, fear of new people)}

Slow comprehension.

— headache from studying.

— homework is an agonising topic for many Tuberculinum youngsters.

— ADD – study is boring. Cannot sit in one place to study.

— poor memory – mistakes in reading, writing.

TUBERCULINUM CONFIRMATORY CHECKLIST

- Grind teeth during sleep.
- Irritable upon awakening.
- Strike their heads.
- Borne with much hair on the scalp and down the spine.
- Misshapen skulls and other birth anomalies, especially on the midline.
- Long Eyelashes.
- Recurrent upper respiratory tract infections.
- Many dental problems, especially too many and badly aligned teeth.
- Swollen and hard cervical glands.
- Chest and lung problems.
- Crave butter, peanut butter.
  Cheese.
  Cold milk.
  Eggs.
  Macaroni.
  Salt.
  Soft, smoked meats, sausages, salami, ham, bacon .
  spicy foods.
  sweets.
  yoghurt.
- Avoid mixed foods.

- Big appetite without weight gain.
- Frequent diarrhoea.
- Bed-wetting.
- Early masturbation.
- Recurrent fevers.
- Family history of tuberculosis of lung problems.
- Aggravation from exposure to animals.

PSYCHO BEHAVIOURIAL CHAR-ACTERISTICS

CHRONIC MIASMS – TUBERCULOSIS

Some practical clinical situations explained:

a. Cases of Mental Retardation associated with Mongolism:

Tuberculinum children are born with a preponderance of congenital anomalies., e.g. Cretinism, Microcephaly, mongolism (Syph, Bar.carb.). Typically puny, backward children as described by Dr. Burnett. The following symptoms if present make selection of Tuberculinum eminent. Other symptoms are patients find it exhausting to apply themselves to a lesson or a project. Some develop headache from studying or concentrating.

b. Home-work:

Home work is an agonising topic for many tubercular youngsters. They may either lie to their parents or they develop physical aggravation such as fatigue, headache.

c. Academic performance:

Many times Tuberculinum child is quite bright and excels in school until befallen with a severe physical illness. The parental description is that "ever since she had pneumonia, she just cannot study."

d. Restlessness:

There is an odd dissatisfaction with whatever he is currently doing tuberculinum children desire to move to change position, to ramble from room to room. This high energy child is hard to keep still and quiet.

e. Travel:

These restless children usually crave for change of location. They love to travel. The most common way this is elicited is by asking about car, bicycle or scooter ride. This is due to the fact that the ride fulfils the inner desire for change.

f. Irritability:

Tuberculinum patients are born irritable and angry, crying and being very fussy, especially upon first awakening. They also exhibit temper tantrums characterised by violence, kicking, scratching others, throwing himself on the ground and shrieking so loud that it is possible to get anything accomplished until he gets his way.

g. Destructive:

Destructiveness in a patient should always make on think of Tuberculinum. There are ample examples in Materia Medica which exhibit self destructive tendency e.g. hitting the head on floor, walls, pulls his hair, picks at his scabs. He is also destructive with others by getting into fights with school mates.

h. Contrariness:

Most of the things which patient is told to do the answer is always negative e.g. arrange your clothes properly the answer is no.

Whenever he is contradicted he becomes angry and violent. This leads to a quarrelsome nature.

I. Changeability:

Moods and behaviour can change quickly. The relatives and friends of the patient often describe the nature as unpredictable. This inconsistency occurs for two reasons; first, the child suffers internally, not really knowing what she wants, yet she knows that she needs something; something other than what she has. The other reason is that the child enjoy being contrary and derives pleasure out of it.

J. Artistic:

The patient shows interest in artistic and musical fields, e.g. during free time the patient in his office or school or in his house scribbles on the paper leisurely which ultimately turns out to be a good piece of art work, without undergoing any basic training in drawing and painting, they have a good sense of artistic ability. At a very young age the patient shows as ability for musical endeavours, e.g. learning to play flute, mouth organ, violin. At the same time day benefit emotionally out of it.

K. Fears

The strongest fear to be seen is a fear of animals, especially cats and dogs and all their wild derivates, e.g. lions, tigers, wolves, bear.

Fear of being alone especially when they are in the dark; fear of new situations, thunderstorms and monsters are also high on the list.

BACILLINUM

SOURCES

The idea of prescribing for a tuberculous patient the sputum of anyone suffering from the same disease, is old.

In 1638, Robert Fludd suggested – 'Sputum rejected from the lungs, after its proper preparation, cures tuberculosis'.

Bacillinum is a nosode of tuberculosis named and first described by Dr. Burnett, for whom it was prepared from tuberculous sputum.

Bacillinum is the maceration of a portion of the lung of an individual who died of pulmonary tuberculosis, containing the bacilli, ptomaine and tubercles in all stages.

In 1854, Dr. Martino from Rio (South America) favoured tubercina (a nosode prepared from a tubercular patient) and called the substance as "Tuberculinum".

Bacillinum must be distinguished from Koch's *Tuberculin*. Bacillinum is a maceration of a typical tuberculous lung. Koch's lymph is an extract in glycerine of dead tuberculous bacilli. The former is compound natural infection; the latter is a product of a laboratory experiment.

MENTAL CHARACTERISTICS

- Tremendous desire for change – begins a task and takes up another even before the first one is finished. Desire to travel.

- Hopefulness. It is seen that even in incurable terminal conditions these patients do not lose hope.

- There is a need to take risks. Fear is not felt to the extent that the situation demands.

- Fear of dogs.

PHYSICAL CHARACTERISTICS

- Of favourable use in chronic non-tubercular disease, when bronchorrhoea and dyspnoea are present.

- Especially indicated in old people, with chronic catarrhal condition and enfeebled pulmonary circulation, with attacks of suffocation at night with difficult cough.

- Cough < raising arms.

    < becoming cold.

    < reading aloud.

    < talking loud.

    < lying on right side.

    < sleep during.

    > in wind.

- Constant disposition to catch colds and sore throats.

74

- Personal or family history of chest affections.
- Favours falling off of tartar from the teeth.
- Talks in sleep. Grinds teeth in sleep. Drowsy during day, restless at night. Many dreams.
- Pain in the head, deep within, worse by motion.
- Abdominal pains, with enlarged glands in the groin. Chronic diarrhoea.
- Ringworm.
- Desires – salt, vinegar, alcohol, eggs, milk, mustard.
- Aversion – chicken, fats, water.
- Aggravation – chicken.

HINTS FOR SPOTTING BACILLINUM ON CLINICAL EXAMINATION

- Alopecia, bald patches of the head and mustache.
- Eczematous condition of the margins of the eyelids.
- Ulcerative eruption on the nose.
- 'Bat-wing' appearance of the junction of nose and check.
- Brownish spots or blotches of the face.
- Strawberry tongue.
- Imperfectly developed teeth.
- Enlargement of cervical lymph nodes.
- Enlarged glands in the groin.
- On auscultation, bubbling rales.

The following symptomatology is extracted from the last edition of Burnett's "The Cure of Consumption by it's own Virus"

RESPIRATORY:

- Congestion of lungs and catarrh of such.
- Oppression, coarse, bubbling rales, purulent expectoration.
- Chronic cough with concomitants of HEAT and SWEAT at night.
- WHEEZING – DYSPNOEA with suffocative attacks at night.
- Old people with chronic catarrhal symptoms and feeble pulmonary circulation.
- Throat studded with tubercles, feverish, expectorates blood and pus.
- Aphonia.
- PHLEGM > A.M.

INDURATED GLANDS:

- Tubercular enlargement of the cervical and mesenteric lymph nodes.
- Look for strumous scar on the neck of the patient indicating removal of tubercular glands.
- Groin full of small indurated glands.

SKIN CONDITIONS:

- Ringworm.
- Ulcerative 'bat-wing' discolouration of nose/cheek junction.
- Alopecia or bald patches of head, mustache.
- Pustular acne without scarring (if pustular and scarring, use Vaccinum or Variolinum)
- Eczematous (redness of eyelid margin)
- Brownish spots/blotches of face.

TUBERCULINUM
(A COMPARISON)

We shall study the comparative materia medica on 2 planes.

1. Physicals
2. Mentals

Physicals

I. TAKES COLD EASILY

A. Arsenic iodide.

This remedy should be thought of when the discharges are acrid, profuse, thick or thin.

A thin watery discharge with burning sensation is a characteristic symptom during the acute attack of cold.

In chronic cases, there is afternoon rise of temperature, yellowish greenish pus like discharge, profound prostration, emaciation, drenching night sweats.

The patient is aggravated in dry cold windy weather and is always better in open air.

B. Calcarea Carbonica:

Calcarea carbonica patients are susceptible to cold

79

damp air; especially the chest is sensitive to cold and hence with slightest exposure to cold the patient develop lower respiratory tract infections with glandular enlargements.

The patient always feels worse when there is change of weather especially from hot to cold.

Patient invariably feels better in a dry climate.

The cold often begins with obstruction of nose, frequent sneezing but with dry nostrils. The tonsils are inflammed and the cold immediately settles in the chest, which is then characterised a cough, felt as a tickling from dust or a feather in the throat. It is worse by inspiration and after eating.

C. Kali Carbonicum:

It is adapted to person who are sensitive to atmospheric changes, to every draft of air, always shivering with a tendency to catch cold.

There is descending coryza with fetid yellow green discharge. There is obstruction of nose which is better by walking in open air, the cold usually leads to dyspnoea.

The expectoration is difficult, yellowish, greenish, offensive with sour and salty taste. Though chilly, the patient feels better in open air.

The respiratory symptoms are worse early morning.

D. Psorinum:

Psorinum is used when well selected remedies fail to relieve or permanently improve or when Sulphur seems indicated but fails.

Weak emaciated individuals who take cold very easily after supression of skin diseases or as ill effect of infectious diseases. There is a history of recurrent quinsy with expectoration of foul, cheesy masses.

The cough returns every winter. It is worse.

Lying down.

Drinking.

Cold drinks.

II.   EATS WELL BUT EMACIATES:

A. Abrotanum

The emaciation of Abrotanum affects mainly the lower extremities. The child is unable to hold the head up due to weakness of neck muscles. There is presence of blue rings around the eyes. The face appears wrinkled and pale. There is marked craving for bread and boiled milk the skin is loose and flabby. There is severe constipation.

B. Iodium:

The characteristic of Iodium emaciation is its rapid progress.

Note: In thyrotoxicosis the patient loses flesh rapidly despite a good appetite. There is presence of great debility; cannot talk, becomes out of breath; the slightest effort produces profuse perspiration.

The emaciation is associated with glandular enlargement and a feeling of internal heat. Clinically it is important to know that along with increased appetite the patient almost always feels better in his physical symptoms by eating. Psychologically the patient gets anxious and worried if he does not eat.

C. Natrum Muriaticum:

The emaciation of Natrum mur is of a descending type, progressing from head to foot. Emaciation is marked near malar bones, neck, clavicles and abdomen. The Natrum Mur emaciation is associated with increased appetite. This increased appetite can be an effect of chronic malaria, silent grief or any reserved displeasure. Patient has desire for salt, bitter things, sour things, farinaceous food, oysters, fish, milk. There is extreme thirst for large quantities of water.

The patient perspires at the margins of the hair (my personal experience in many cases).

III. HUNGRY GETS UP AT NIGHTS TO EAT:

A. Cinchona:

The debility, emaciation and anaemia forces an element of voracious appetite, especially in those who are previously emaciated. As soon as he eats a little there is a sensation of heavy weight in the stomach and the voracious appetite is marked. They always want to eat sweets with every meal; even waking up at night to raid the refrigerator to satisfy their craving.

B. Lycopodium:

In Lycopodium, it is the sluggish function of the liver and gall bladder which is responsible for various G.I.T. complaints. The weakness, and emaciation forces the patient to develop a canine appetite; the more he eats the more he craves. That is the reason why he wakes up in the night feeling hungry, eats a little which creates a fullness in the abdomen and there is excessive formation of flatulence and pressure around the abdomen. There is craving for sweets and farinaceous food, and cabbage and oysters which puts his digestive system out of gear.

IV. DESIRES SMOKED MEAT:

This signifies that the patient has marked desire for smoked beef and various other salted meats.

A. Causticum:

Fresh meat causes nausea and hence to satisfy the desire of eating meat the patient craves smoked meat to such an extent that he prefers to have it at every meal without any additives.

Sometimes after its consumption the patient develops a continuous salty taste in the mouth for a long time.

B. Kreosote:

Indicated in emaciated under-developed children who have food fads, especially for smoked meats. This craving is also seen in terminally ill cancer patients who vomit every kind of food but retain smoked meat.

V. DESIRES REFRESHING THINGS:

Phosophoric Acid:

The appetite of Acid Phos patients is extremely poor due to severe mental and physical debility. There is severe distension and fermentation in bowels; hence such a condition. Patient is unable to take solid foods, heavy foods, as he immediately gets some risings. Instead there is a strong craving for Juicy refreshing things (fresh juice, canned juice, cold milk).

VI. DESIRES COLD MILK

Rhus Toxicodendron:

Rhus Tox patient is extremely thirsty without having any appetite for any kind of food. Patient is extremely chilly. Cold in any form aggravates, especially the cough, but with this exists a strong desire for cold milk. Patient relishes it even though it may aggravate the cough.

VII. DESIRES HIGHLY SEASONED FOOD

Syphilinum:

The patient has a capricious appetite which is characterized by craving for alcoholic liquors. When he wants to eat a substantial meal he wants it extremely spicy even though there are ulcers in the mouth and teeth are decayed.

VIII. DESIRES FAT

Nitric Acid:

There is a ravenous appetite which cannot be satisfied with plain food. Hence patient develops the habit of adding fat to food which gives them a sense of satisfaction. It is so peculiar that fats are consumed here with salt; e.g. butter, ghee. However, patient has a strong aversion to sweets. Hence any combination of fat and sweets in rejected by the patient e.g. sweetmeats.

IX. AVERSION TO MEAT:

Sanicula:

The aversion for meat in a Sanicula patient is only partial as the patient has marked desire for bacon. The patient is extremely thirsty, drinks little and often; yet is undernourished.

X. AVERSION TO SMELL OF COFFEE:

Lachesis:

It is only the odour of coffee which aggravates the patient as such the patient has desire for coffee.

Thirsty but fears to drink because of the sensation of chocking.

XI.   NODES IN BREAST:

Conium:

Breast enlarged and painful before and during menses, worse at every step, the patient wants to press the breast hard with both hands.

Hard tumours in Mammae with stitching or piercing pain.

XII.   GLANDULAR ENLARGEMENT:

Bacillinum:

The patient has constant disposition to take cold. Glands of the neck are enlarged and tender.

The patient is extremely chilly and sensitive to draft and cold air.

XIII.   EARLY MORNING DIARRHOEA:

Sulphur:

The patient has hurry to the toilet. Diarrhoea is painless, watery and offensive, worse after milk.

XIV.   GRINDS TEETH IN SLEEP:

Cina:

Night terrors of children, cries out, screams, wakes up frightened. Screams and talks in sleep.

Grinds teeth in sleep.

86

INDICATIONS OF UNCOMMON AND COMMON REMEDIES USED IN TUBERCULAR CONDITIONS

Acalypha India

Incipient phthisis with hard, hacking cough, bloody expectoration, bright red haemoptysis. Blood bright red and not profuse in morning, dark and clotted in afternoon.

Agaricin

An Active constituent of polyporus officinate – phthisical and other enervating night sweats.

Agraphis Nutans

Catarrhs obstruction, adenoid. Tendency to take cold.

Allium Sativa

Pulmonary T.B. Patients who eat a lot. Rattling of mucus and rhonchi; Cough in the morning on leaving the room. Darting pain in chest. Expectoration dark difficult.

Alumina

Haemoptysis with weakness of chest. Copious expectoration, especially in the morning. Induration of gland with tendency to ulceration.

Antimony-iodide

Pneumonia and bronchitis.
Loss of strength and appetite;
Sweat profuse.
Chronic colds which are extended downwards.
Hard cough with wheeze and inability to raise the sputum.

Balsam peruvianum

Bronchial catarrh.
Copious purulent expectoration.
Loose cough with hectic fever.
Irritating, short cough.

Baryta Carbonica

Dry, suffocative cough especially of old people. Chest is full of mucus but lacking strength to expectorate.
Beta-vulgaris
Chronic catarrhal states and Tuberculosis.

Blatta Orientalis

Cough with dyspnoea in bronchitis phthisis
Much pus like mucus.

Boletus Laricus

Night sweats in Tuberculosis
Hectic fever.

Calcarea-carbonica

Incipient phthisis — Expectoration-thick,
Tickling cough — Sour mucus
Fleeting chest pains — Cough night
Dislike for fat — Chest very sensitive to touch, percussion & pressure.

Gets out of breath easily
Increased sweating which — Bloody expectoration
is cold and sour with sour sensation in chest.

Calcarea-iodide

Scrofulous affection.
Affects glands.
Flabby children subject to colds.
Chronic cough.
Hectic fever.
Green, purulent expectoration.

Calcarea – fluorica

Cough with expectoration of tiny lumps of yellow mucus with tickling cough and irritation worse on lying down; Exhausting night sweats; Bleeding from lungs.

Calcarea-Phosphorica

Anaemia with tuberculosis-Cough lying down
Swollen glands.

Profuse perspiration.

Hoarseness of voice.

Calcarea – Silicata

Sensitive to cold

Chilly patient but worse on being overheated.

Emaciated.

Pain in the chest with copious, yellow, green mucus.

Calotropis

Pneumonic Phthisis.

T.B. of the syphilitic miasm if mercury cannot be used any further.

Obesity.

Heat in stomach.

Anaemia.

Carbo-veg.

Burning in the chest with haemoptysis.

Spasmodic cough with gagging and vomiting of mucus.

Hoarseness, worse evening.

Haemorrhage from lung.

Hectic fever with exhausting sweats.

Cetraria

Phthisis with bloody expectoration.

China-arsenicum

Weariness and sudden prostration.
Dyspnoea with profuse sweat.

Drosera

Drosera can break resistance to tubercle and therefor should be capable of raising it – Tyler.

Spasmodic T.B. cough, worse evening lying down, worse midnight, worse getting warm in bed, worse drinking, singing, laughing.

Spasmodic, dry, cough – in paroxysms which follow each other rapidly.

Expectoration yellow.

Bleeding from nose & mouth.

Retching – sensation – crumbs were in the throat, or feather in the larynx.

Laryngeal phthisis with rapid emaciation–phthisis Pulmonum and tubercular glands.

Eriodictyon

Chronic bronchitis with bronchial tuberculosis with profuse easily raised bronchial secretions. Dull pain in right lung.

Bronchial phthisis with night sweats and emaciation.

Furthers absorption of effusion in pleural cavity.

Ferrum arsenicum

Phthisis with enlarged liver and spleen, pernicious anaemia.

Ferrum Phosphoricum

In acute exacerbation of T.B. – palliative wonderful power.

Congestion of lungs – haemoptysis – Expectoration of pure blood.

Hard dry cough with sore chest, better night.

Corresponds to Grauvogl's Oxygenoid constitution – The inflammatory febrile, emaciating wasting consumptive.

Ficus religiosa

Difficulty in breathing.

Cough.

Haemoptysis, haemorrhage arrester.

Formic acid

Tuberculosis with subacute and chronic nephritis and chronic arthritis.

Formica rufa

Tendency to take cold.

Tuberculosis.

Hoarseness with dry sore throat.

Cough worse night with aching in forehead and constrictive pain in the chest.

Pleuritic pains.

Guaiacol

Pleuritic pains.

Hippozaenium

Tuberculosis with chronic cavity in lung, Excessive expectoration producing noisy breathing.

Inula

Palliative in Tubercular laryngitis. Teasing cough with much and free expectoration.

Iodoform

Tuberculous condition especially used in Tubercular meningitis. Cough and wheezing on going to bed with haemoptysis, chronic diarrhoea in Tubercular constitution.

Manganum

T. B. of Larynx, Chronic hoarseness.

Cough worse evening.

Better lying down.

Great accumulation of mucus.

Soreness, aching Haemoptysis.

Every cold arouses bronchitis. Nose dry obstructed.

Medorrhinum

Incipient T. B. Sore Larynx. Chronic nasal and pharyngeal catarrhs. Hectic night sweats.

Craves liquor, salts, sweets. Throat is sore and swollen. Deglutition of liquids or solids is impossible. Throat constantly filled with thick grey bloody mucus from posterior nares. Incessant dry cough at night.

Iodium

Emaciation with great appetite. General debility. Enlarged lymphatic glands. Nasal engorgement.

Goitre

Acute affections of the respiratory organs.

Kali-carbonicm:

Tubercular diathesis, irritable.

Obstinate

Hypersensitive.

Nose stuffs up in a warm room. Hoarseness.

Stitching pains in chest, better leaning forwards.

Cough up cheesy lumps.

Recurrent colds.

Kali nitricum

Debility and relapse in T.B. Hoarseness. Expectorates clotted blood after hawking.

Lachnanthes

Early stages of T.B. and established chest cases. Loquacity. Circumscribed red cheeks. Tendency to sweat. Septic throats.

Lactic acid

Tubercular ulceration of vocal cords as of a lump in the throat, keeps swallowing.

Lycopodium

Tubercular laryngitis especially when ulceration starts. Tickling cough. Dyspnoea.

Expectoration thick, grey, bloody, purulent, salty. Constriction of chest, burning in chest. Stitches and dryness of throat, better warm drinks. Stuffed up nose. Snuffles, fluent coryza, ulcerated nostrils, crusts.

Myositis

Chronic bronchitis and phthisis. Night sweats, cough with profuse muco-purulent expectoration, gagging and vomiting during cough, worse while or after eating. Bronchorrhoea. Pain in left lung; pain while coughing and sensitive to percussion.

Myrtus communis

Chest pains as often found in consumption. Dry hollow cough Tickling.

Naphthaline

Pulmonary T.B., Gonorrhoea, whooping cough, Terrible offensive ammoniacal urine. Acute Laryngo-tracheitis. Tenacious expectoration. Hay fever.

Natrum – selenium

Laryngeal phthisis with expectoration of small lumps of bloody mucus and slight hoarseness.

Nitric-acid

Hoarseness, aphonia, with dry hacking cough, from tickling in larynx and pit of stomach, soreness at lower end of sternum. Short breath on going upstairs. Cough during sleep.

Oleum santali

2-3 drops on sugar will frequently relieve hacking cough when but little sputum is expectorated.

Oxalic Acid

Nervous aphonia with cardiac derangement. Burning sensation from throat down. Hoarseness. Left lung painful. Aphonia. Dyspnoea, short jerking inspirations.

Sharp pain through lower region of left lung extending down to epigastrium.

Phellandrium

A very good remedy for offensive expectoration and cough in phthisis, bronchitis and emphysema. Tuberculosis affecting generally middle lobes.

Haemoptysis, hectic and colliquative diarrhoea. Cough with profuse and fetid expectoration, compels him to sit up.

Hoarseness.

Phosphorus

T.B. Haemoptysis, incipient and more advanced T.B. Oppression of chest. Rusty sputum. Hoarseness.

Pain in larynx. Tightness in chest-as of a weight. Heat in chest. Tickling cough worse cold air, talking, Sweetish taste

Pilocarpus

Bronchial mucous membrane inflammed. Much inclination to cough and difficult breathing. Oedema of lungs. Foamy sputa. Profuse, thin serous expectoration. Slow respiration.

Polygonus aviculare

Phthisis pulmonalis and intermittent fever.

Salvia

Phthisis with night-sweats and suffocating tickling cough. Tickling cough, especially in consumption.

Silicea

Cough fails to yield, sputum persistently muco-purulent and profuse. Slow recovery after pneumonia. Cough with expectoration in day, bloody or purulent. Stitches in chest through to back. Violent cough when lying down with thick yellow lumpy expectoration, suppurative stage of expectoration.

Spongia

The dry chronic sympathetic cough of organic heart disease is relieved by Spongia.

Cough-dry, barking, croupy. Larynx sensitive to touch.

Worse during inspiration, before midnight. Respiration short, panting, difficult sensation of plug in larynx. Cough abates after eating or drinking especially warm drinks. Laryngeal phthisis.

Stannum Metallicum

T.B. Hectic fever. Weakness. Copious, green, sweet expectoration. Cough excited by laughing and talking chest weak and can hardly talk. Exhausting night sweats especially towards morning.

Teucrium scorodonia:

Tuberculosis with muco-purulent expectoration, dropsy, orchitis and tuberculous epididymitis, especially in young, thin individuals with T.B. of lungs, glands, bones and uro-genitals.

TUBERCULAR MIASM, DIATHE-SIS AND DYSCRASIA

TUBERCULAR MIASM

I am extremely grateful to late Dr. M.L. Dhawale, whose symposium volumes were my basis of understanding the above miasm. He mentions that tubercular constitution is characterised by symptoms that resemble negative nitrogen balance. Emaciation, thus, is a strong feature of this miasm.

All the characteristics of psoric phase that are present are strongly enhanced. Eg., a simple itch due to a small vesicle may now suppurate with pain and itching which is uncontrollable; also a bland nasal discharge due to irritation of strong odours now secondarily gets infected and turns purulent.

It is very important to know that a simple inflammation under the influence of tubercular miasm, turns into suppuration and ultimately the repair takes place, either by ulceration or fibrosis. Also hypertrophy, enlargement and atrophy are very common glandular involvements under this miasm. The person is strongly preoccupied with sex, sexual fantasies and other lascivious traits. Changeability or too short interest are other peculiarities

99

of this miasm, eg., change in profession, change in relationships, change in sexual partners.

Also falling into this miasm are various 'Aberrant Immune Responses' which are directed towards 'self, eg., Rheumatoid arthritis, Ankylosing Spondylitis.

TUBERCULAR DIATHESIS

To understand diathesis, one has to understand what is constitution. A healthy constitution is indicative of maximal stability under given environmental circumstances and the inherited reactivity.

Diathesis is an abnormal constitution with expression of susceptibility under strain. This strain is generally inherited by the strong influences of certain diseases and traits that run in families, through generations, Eg., a strong history of pulmonary tuberculosis in parents, grandparents and siblings, make a person develop tubercular diathesis.

TUBERCULAR DYSCRASIA

Dyscrasia means a defect that remains in the constitution after the removal of the disease state Eg., after suffering from pulmonary tuberculosis, a person has become highly prone to recurrent respiratory tract infection or after suffering from Abdominal Koch's a person is highly prone to excessive generation of flatus. According to principle of Homoeopathic Philosophy, treating an infection with antibiotics and other chemotherapeutic agents will definitely remove the symptoms but without changing the susceptibility and hence the person is extremely prone to recurrence. Unfortunately, in diseases like tuberculosis, Homeopathic literature lacks evidence of cases cured purely with Homoeopathic medicines. I am very honest to declare that even in my personal practice, I have no evidence of treating, purely with Homoeopathic medicines, any case of tuberculosis in any organ of the body.

TREATMENT FOR TUBERCULAR MIASM

To treat any miasmatic disorder, one has to consider the give miasm under the following titles.

1. Predisposition: Persons who are predisposed to develop illness resembling tuberculosis or developing tuberculosis or suffering from symptoms which are indicative of tubercular miasm have strong history of (a) tuberculosis anywhere in the body (b) either in parents or grandparents or 1st cousins.

    This is what we commonly call FUNDAMENTAL CAUSE.

2. Expression: By expression I mean constitution; i.e. a person having TUBERCULAR DIATHESIS.

    Tubercular diathesis should be suspected in an individual who has following signs and symptoms.

    Opening doors-e.g. if in a given case one has a history of any tubercular illness like pulmonary kochs, fibrosis of lung, recurrent pneumonia, recurrent tubercular lymphadenitis and the patient is really never well since then, in such condition one can always start with either tuberculinum or Bacillinum.

3. Obstacles to Recovery : In certain cases when the indicated drug does not give adequate response or fails to act and one finds tubercular miasm as a strong dominant feature, one can always use it as an intercurrent remedy.

4. As an acute prescription : Late Dr. Sarabhai Kapadia and late Dr. Maganlal Desai had in the past treated cases of acute tubercular meningitis and acute pulmonary tuberculosis with either Tuberculinum or Bacillinum.

5. Prophylaxis: Dr. Kent has mentioned that Tuberculinum should be used as a prophylactic medicine in children with a strong family history of tuberculosis.

6. Lingering illness: Any lingering condition having a tubercular background e.g. a pneumonia with a tubercular background requires tuberculinum (as against pneumonia with a sycotic background which requires Nat. sulph:)

TUBERCULINUM IN VERSES

Suitable to persons of tuberculous diathesis who are physically weak but mentally precocious;

Who have tall, slim, flat, narrow chests, blue eyes, blonde in preference to burnettes;

When there is a family history of tuberculosis & drugs you have tried with all your resources;

But nothing cures permanently or fails to relieve One can try Tuberculinum without reference to name of disease;

Symptoms keep on changing from one organ to another To lungs, brain, kidneys, stomach or liver;

All of a sudden the symptoms just crop and without any notice they also drop;

Takes cold easily without knowing how or where, Seems to take cold every time he breathes fresh air;

Eats very well but rapidly emaciates as if the food in stomach simply evaporates;

Melancholic morose, irritable & sulky basically sweet, now running towards insanity;

Everything in the room looks so strange as if the things there have undergone a change;

Deep tuberculous headache & intense neuralgia
Crops of painful boils & Plica Polonica;

School girl's headache worse by mental study. Acts
best in a case with a tubercular history;

Tuberculous meningitis with threatened effusion.
Wake up frightened from hallucination;

Diarrhoea early morning sudden & imperative,
stool dark brown, watery & offensive;

Menses too early, too profuse, too long lasting with
frightful dysmenorrhoea but tardy in starting;

Eczema tubercular over entire body Intensely itching & heavily scaly;

Craving for cold milk & aversion to meat. All-gone
hungry feeling that drives him to eat;

Desire for open air & a change of place. As if in
sight-seeing he is running a race.

{Verses written by Late Dr. Kirpal Singh Bakshi}

BIBLIOGRAPHY

1. **REPERTORY OF THE HOMOEOPATHIC MATERIA MEDICA** BY.J.T.KENT A.M., M.D
   ENRICHED INDIAN EDITION, REPRINTED SIXTH AMERICAN EDITION

2. **SYNTHETIC REPERTORY PSYCHIC AND GENERAL SYMPTOMS OF THE HOMOEOPATHIC MATERIA MEDIA**
   PUBLISHED BY: DR. MED HORST WILHEMSFEELD

3. **THE PRACTICE OF HOMOEOPATHY, NOTES ON THE NOSODES**
   TUBERCULINUM AND BACILLINUM BY SHEILAGH CREASY, BAFA, RS HOM

4. **THERAPEUTIC OF THE RESPIRATORY ORGANS** BY FRANCOIS CARTIER, M.D.

5. **TREATISE ON DYNAMISED MICRO IMMUNOTHERAPY** BY O.A. JULIAN
   TRANSLATED BY: RAJKUMAR MUKERJI

6. **PORTRAITS OF HOMOEOPATHIC MEDICINES PSYCHOPHYSICAL ANALYSES OF SELECTED CONSTITUTIONAL TYPES.**
   BY CATHERINE R. COULTER

7. **HOMOEOPATHIC DRUG PICTURES** BY DR. M.L. TYLER

8. **LECTURES ON HOMOEOPATHIC MATERIA MEDICA** BY J.T. KENT

9. **A DICTIONARY OF PRACTICAL MATERIA MEDICA** BY J.H.CLARKE

10. **AN INTRODUCTION TO PRINCIPLES AND PRACTICE OF HOMOEOPATHY** BY CHARLES E. WHEELER M.D., B.Sc. (LOND.)